BREAST CARE

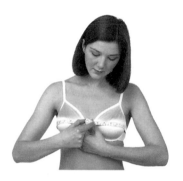

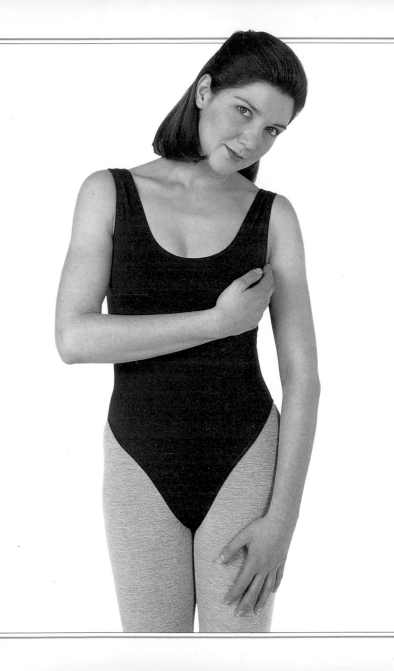

ESSENTIAL TIPS

BREAST CARE

Dr. Miriam Stoppard

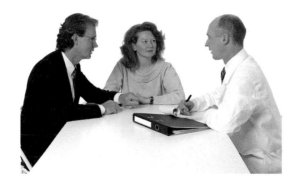

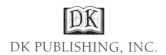

DK PUBLISHING, INC.

A DK PUBLISHING BOOK

Editor Alison Copland
Art Editor Bill Mason
Senior Editor Gillian Roberts
Series Art Editor Alison Donovan
Production Controller Hélène Lamassoure
US Editor Laaren Brown

First American Edition, 1997
2 4 6 8 10 9 7 5 3 1
Published in the United States by DK Publishing, Inc.
95 Madison Avenue, New York, New York 10016

Visit us on the World Wide Web at http://www.dk.com

A catalog record is available from the Library of Congress

ISBN 0-7894-1975-0

Text film output by The Right Type, Great Britain
Reproduced by Colourscan, Singapore
Printed and bound in Italy by Graphicom

ESSENTIAL TIPS

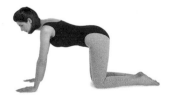

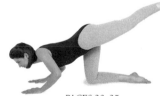

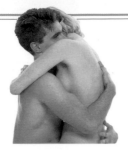

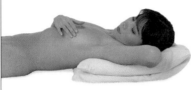

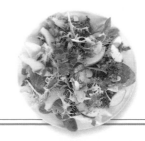

WHAT ARE BREASTS?

1 THE FEMALE BODY

Women's bodies vary greatly in shape and size, but all tend toward one of the three main body types: endomorph (apple-shaped), mesomorph (pear-shaped), and ectomorph (beanpole-shaped). The basic body structure can always be identified, although its contours, including the breasts, may be altered through diet and exercise.

THE IDEAL SHAPE
Throughout the world, popular ideas of the perfect shape for a woman's body vary widely. In some cultures, a full, plump figure is regarded as highly desirable, whereas others place more importance on a slim, athletic figure.

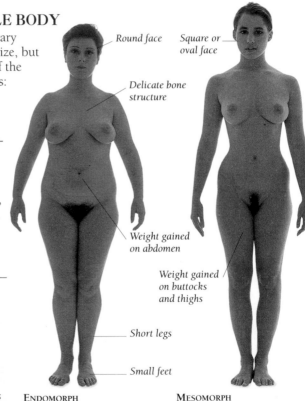

Round face

Square or oval face

Delicate bone structure

Weight gained on abdomen

Weight gained on buttocks and thighs

Short legs

Small feet

ENDOMORPH
Breasts tend to be larger than average, and weight is gained easily.

MESOMORPH
Legs are same length as torso, hips larger than shoulders, and breasts average in size.

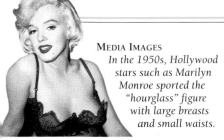

MEDIA IMAGES
In the 1950s, Hollywood stars such as Marilyn Monroe sported the "hourglass" figure with large breasts and small waists.

2 POSITION OF THE BREASTS

The breasts lie outside the rib cage and the pectoral muscles covering the chest. They extend vertically from the second to the sixth rib, horizontally from the breast bone across the rib cage, and into the armpit (the axillary tail). The breasts merge with the body fat around them, except where they extend to the armpits and pierce the muscles of the chest wall.

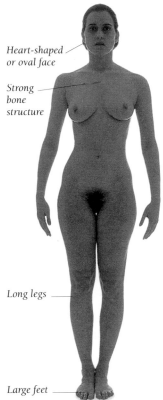

Heart-shaped or oval face

Strong bone structure

Long legs

Large feet

ECTOMORPH
Legs are longer than torso, and breasts may be small. Weight is evenly distributed over the body and is not gained easily.

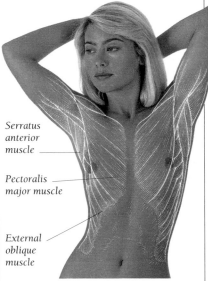

Serratus anterior muscle

Pectoralis major muscle

External oblique muscle

POSITION ON THE MUSCLES
The interior surface of the breast lies closely against the muscles of the chest, most especially the pectoralis major, but to a lesser extent the serratus anterior and the external oblique.

3 BREAST ANATOMY

The breasts are simply highly modified sweat glands, but ones that secrete milk rather than sweat. They consist of glandular elements – the milk-producing lobes and ducts – and the connective tissue that forms the supporting structure. The lobes are subdivided into lobules. Toward the nipple, each duct widens to form a sac, or ampulla. A layer of fat surrounding the glandular tissue cushions the breasts.

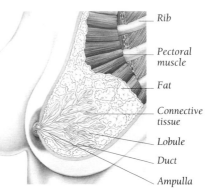

Rib

Pectoral muscle

Fat

Connective tissue

Lobule

Duct

Ampulla

INSIDE THE BREAST
The glandular tissue, the working part of the breast, is protected by fat. The amount of fat determines the size and shape of the breast. The ratio of fat to glandular tissue tends to increase with age.

4 BLOOD SUPPLY

Arteries carry oxygen-rich blood from the heart to the chest wall and breasts, and veins take deoxygenated blood back to the heart. The axillary artery passes from the armpit and supplies the outer half of the breast, while the internal mammary artery comes from the neck and supplies the inner half. Veins from the breast take blood back to the heart via those of the armpit and rib spaces, and then into veins deeper within the chest. A network of veins also connects with the main external jugular vein, and then drains into the heart.

Axillary artery

Branches of the internal mammary artery

ARTERIES & VEINS
Blood reaches the breast via arteries, and then returns to the heart through veins.

5 THE NIPPLE & AREOLA

Nipples can be flat, round, conical, or cylindrical. The color is determined by the thinness and pigmentation of the nipple's skin; whether the nipple is soft or firm depends on the tone of the muscle fibers located within it. The dark, flat area surrounding the nipple itself is known as the areola.

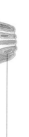

Duct
Hair
Areola muscle
Tubercle of Montgomery
Sebaceous gland

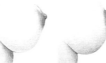

FLAT NIPPLE   ERECT NIPPLE

◁ **NIPPLE RESPONSE**
The nipple is surrounded by tiny muscles that respond to stimulation. When these contract, the areola puckers and the nipple becomes hard and elongated.

◁ **CROSS-SECTION**
The nipple and areola contain sweat glands, hair follicles, and sebaceous glands, which secrete a lubricating substance called sebum.

THE AREOLA
The skin of the areola is very thin, and its surface is marked by small bumps known as the tubercles of Montgomery.

6 BREAST FUNCTION

Accessories to the main organs of reproduction, breasts provide essential milk for the newborn baby and also play an important part in sexual activity. Men's breasts have the same basic structure as women's, and male nipples can be equally sensitive. In puberty, a slight hormone imbalance may cause boys to develop tiny breasts.

BREASTS IN OLDER MEN
Obvious breasts may develop, as lower levels of the male hormone testosterone allow the female estrogen to dominate.

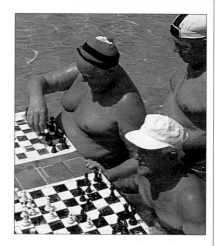

11

HOW BREASTS DEVELOP

7 IN THE WOMB

Breast development begins very early in the embryo. At about six weeks, there is a thickening of the skin called the mammary ridge, or milk line. By six months, this extends from the armpit to the groin, but dies back, leaving two breast buds on the upper half of the chest. In a female, columns of cells then grow inward from each bud, and become separate sweat or exocrine glands, with ducts leading to the nipple, before birth.

MALE & FEMALE
The earliest stages of breast development are identical in male and female fetuses. Men could develop fully functioning breasts, given the right hormonal conditions.

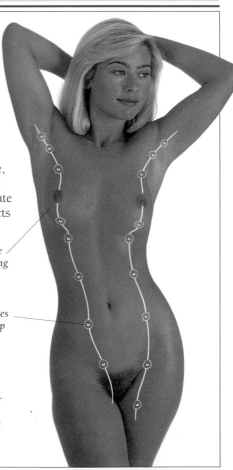

Normal site of developing breasts

Extra nipples may develop anywhere along milk line

ALONG THE MILK LINE
This is a common site for extra nipples or rudimentary breasts, which may persist into adult life; more rarely, the two breast buds fade away with the rest of the milk line, so that nipples are absent at birth.

8 EFFECTS OF HORMONE ACTIVITY

Throughout a woman's life, her breasts are influenced by hormones, which cause changes in size and shape, especially during puberty, and monthly changes in her fertile years. Some women feel premenstrual tenderness or pain in the breasts because of these changes. Hormonal activity lessens after menopause.

HORMONE RECEPTORS
Breasts contain millions of receptor cells, which respond to hormones. Their sensitivity varies from woman to woman.

THE MONTHLY CYCLE
Before menopause, estrogen and progesterone are active throughout the monthly cycle. Progesterone is absent from the onset of menopause, and estrogen production gradually declines.

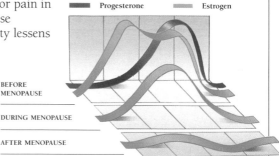

Progesterone   Estrogen

BEFORE MENOPAUSE

DURING MENOPAUSE

AFTER MENOPAUSE

9 WHAT HAPPENS DURING PUBERTY?

At the age of 10 or 11, the first external signs of developing breasts appear. As the ovaries begin to secrete estrogen, fat accumulates in the connective tissue of the breasts and causes them to enlarge. The duct system also begins to develop at this stage, but the mechanism that secretes milk does not develop until pregnancy.

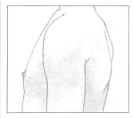

1 Before puberty, the breast is flat except for the nipple protruding from the areola.

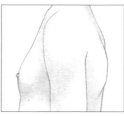

2 As puberty starts, the areola becomes a prominent bud and the breast begins to fill out.

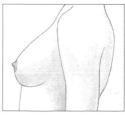

3 Glandular tissue and fat within the breast increase, and the areola eventually flattens out.

10 THE MATURE BREAST

During puberty, secretory glands at the ends of the milk ducts are formed, and with further growth, the lobes of the glands become separated by dense connective tissue and fat deposits. This stretchy tissue allows for enlargement during pregnancy when the glandular elements swell.

Breast development is not really complete until a woman has given birth and breast-fed her baby, during which time additional changes occur (*Tips 36–44*).

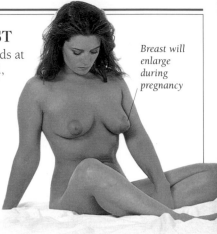

Breast will enlarge during pregnancy

11 CHANGES DURING MENSTRUATION

Each month, a fertile woman undergoes fluctuations in hormone levels as part of the menstrual cycle. In the days just before her period, this can cause her breasts to enlarge and become tender. Nipples may become sensitive or painful.

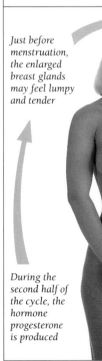

Just before menstruation, the enlarged breast glands may feel lumpy and tender

In the first half of the menstrual cycle, the ovaries produce estrogen

During the second half of the cycle, the hormone progesterone is produced

Halfway through the cycle, the increasing estrogen leads to ovulation

ALLEVIATING PAIN
Tenderness or pain in the breasts a few days before menstruation can some-times be alleviated by the use of evening primrose oil (avoid in pregnancy) or other alternative treatments (Tip 60).

12 MENOPAUSE & BEYOND

During menopause, there is a reduction in estrogen stimulation to all tissues of the body, including the breast tissue, causing the breasts gradually to sag and flatten. Breast tenderness and pain, called mastalgia, can also occur at this time and can sometimes be relieved by using evening primrose oil.

In some women, menopause can bring with it an enormous increase in the size of their breasts, possibly as a result of unregulated estrogen activity.

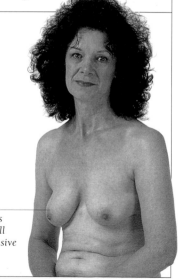

Breast starts to flatten

Glandular tissue reduces

BEYOND MENOPAUSE

After the completion of menopause, a woman's breasts are still capable of responding positively to sexual and other stimuli, despite any physical changes that have taken place.

LOSS OF FULLNESS

In most menopausal women, as estrogen production declines, the glandular tissue of the breasts is reduced, causing the breasts to lose their fullness and begin to sag.

13 THE AGING BREAST

Although the body generally shows signs of wear as it ages, the breasts do not undergo any additional significant physical changes. There is no reason why they should be any more susceptible to disease at this time than at any other. This is especially true if you adopt a positive outlook to aging, and continue to follow a healthy and active lifestyle, making the most of your later years.

A HEALTHY BODY

There is no reason why you can't enjoy reasonable physical fitness well into retirement, and every woman should continue to take sensual pleasure in her body.

Older breasts are still responsive

SIZE, SHAPE & SUPPORT

14 WHAT IS "NORMAL"?

Many women think that their breasts are not "normal," because of recurrent media and advertising images that portray the ideal breast as pert, rounded, firm, and hairless. The truth is that all female breasts have a primary function – to produce milk – and are normal, whatever their size or shape. What is important is that you should feel comfortable and happy with your body.

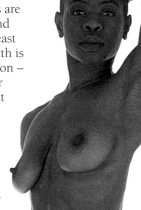

PHYSICAL TYPE
Breast shape is not affected by a woman's basic body type (Tip 1).

MEDIA IMAGE
A slim, firm figure may conform to media ideals, but all breasts are "normal."

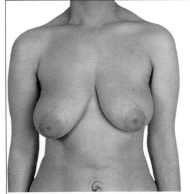

15 ASYMMETRY

A woman's breasts are very rarely entirely symmetrical, but in most cases the difference is of little concern. If you find it disconcerting, however, you can have surgery to correct the imbalance, either by reducing the larger breast or enlarging the smaller one (*Tip 100*).

OBVIOUS DIFFERENCE
One breast may be significantly larger than the other, and may be heavier and sit lower on the chest than the smaller one.

16 SMALL OR FLAT BREASTS

Breasts are measured in terms of chest circumference (in inches or centimeters) and fullness (cup sizes AA–EE). You may have small or flat breasts; this need not be a cause for concern. You are just as capable of breast-feeding a baby as any other woman, and your breasts may fill out during pregnancy and lactation.

SHAPE & POSITION
Small breasts tend to be apple shaped, and they are light in weight. They stand high and pert, and are positioned well away from the chest wall.

THE YOUTHFUL BREAST
A small breast is a youthful breast that will droop and flatten with time.

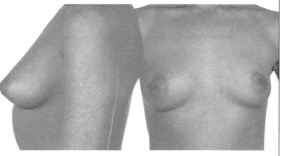

AVERAGE CIRCUMFERENCE, SMALL CUP SIZE

17 LARGE BREASTS

The great variety in size and shape of the breast stems from the layer of subcutaneous fat that surrounds the nipple. If well supported, large breasts need not cause any problems. If the size and weight of your breasts causes you discomfort, however, a breast reduction operation (*Tip 97*) might be worth considering.

SHAPE & POSITION
Large breasts tend to be melon shaped. They are relatively heavy, and this causes them to hang down and lie close to the chest wall.

FURTHER CHANGES
Breasts become more pendulous during and after pregnancy.

LARGE CIRCUMFERENCE, EXTRA-LARGE CUP SIZE

18 BREAST DENSITY AT DIFFERENT AGES

As a woman grows older, the glandular tissue in her breasts becomes less dense. This is one of the reasons why mammography is more effective as a screening technique for older women – in young women, the density of the tissue masks any abnormal shadows on the image. Other screening methods such as ultrasound are used in young women at risk of breast cancer.

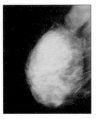 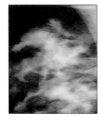 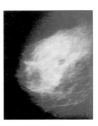 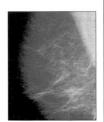

AGE UNDER 30
Only the glandular tissue (the white area) shows up.

AGE 30 TO 40
Darker areas of fatty tissue show around the white.

AGE MID-40S
The glandular tissue continues to reduce in density.

AGE OVER 55
Glandular tissue is a fine network over the darker areas.

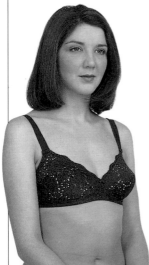

19 WHY WEAR A BRA?

A bra that fits well can make you feel more comfortable, enhance your appearance, and, in the long run, help keep your breasts from sagging. In fact, wearing a bra is one of the best things you can do for your breasts. As a teenager, you should begin wearing a bra as soon as there's any weight in your breasts, especially if you are active in sports. The earlier you wear your first bra, the better.

FEELING COMFORTABLE
If your breasts feel very full and tender in the second half of your menstrual cycle, wear a soft-cup bra for extra comfort at that time.

CAUTION
If you don't wear a bra, especially during exercise, the suspensory ligaments that hold the breasts may become stretched.

20 MEASURING FOR A BRA

Measure your rib cage underneath your breasts, then the fullest part of your bust. For your bra back size, add 4in (10cm) to an even ribcage measurement, 5in (12cm) to an odd one.

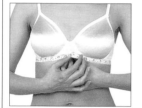

WHAT CUP SIZE?
If the difference between the two measurements is up to 5in (12cm), you are a size A cup; 6in (15cm), size B; 7in (18cm), size C; and so on.

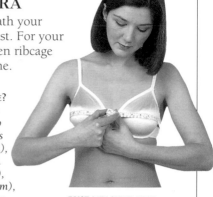

RIB CAGE MEASUREMENT

BUST MEASUREMENT

21 DIFFERENT TYPES OF BRAS

There are many types of bras available. Underwire bras include push-up and minimizer bras that alter breast shape, and long-line, strapless, and half-cup bras for wearing under evening dresses. Soft-cup bras can often be more practical and comfortable for everyday wear, and there are also special nursing and sports bras.

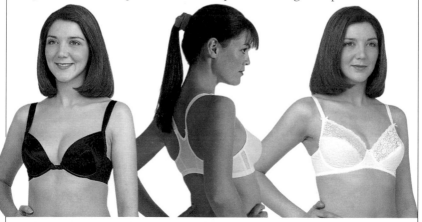

△ PUSH-UP BRA   △ SPORTS BRA   △ UNDERWIRE BRA

A HEALTHY LIFESTYLE

22 EAT A BALANCED DIET

To maintain your general health and fitness, eat a range of different foods every day to satisfy your nutritional needs. Choose something from each of the five main food groups: bread, cereals, and other grain products; fruit; vegetables; meat, poultry, fish, eggs, plant protein sources such as beans; and dairy products.

FRESH FRUIT
A huge range of fresh fruits is now available all year round. Many are a good source of dietary fiber and vitamins, especially A, C, and beta-carotene, which help with cell regeneration.

VEGETABLES & SALADS
Eating plenty of vegetables and salads every day will boost your intake of the essential vitamins, minerals, and fiber that your body needs.

SOURCES OF PROTEIN
Protein is an important part of a healthy diet, helping the formation of new cells and maintaining healthy tissues. It is found not just in lean meat but also in fish, legumes, eggs, dairy products, and whole grains.

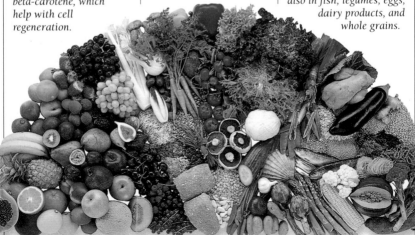

23 IS IT SAFE TO DRINK ALCOHOL?

In moderation, drinking alcohol is safe, and it has even been suggested that it may provide some health benefits. Always remember, however, that alcohol is potentially an addictive drug, and consumed in excess can have very harmful effects on the liver (occasionally indirectly causing breast cancer), the heart, and the brain.

ALCOHOL AND THE RISK FOR BREAST CANCER
Moderate drinking of about one drink per day is not a great risk for breast cancer. Only one extra case of breast cancer per 1,000 women will develop from moderate drinking.

HARD LIQUOR

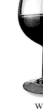
WINE

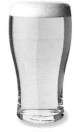
BEER

24 SMOKING

Most people know that smoking can cause lung cancer and heart disease, but they may not know that it may also provoke breast problems. Complications related to ectasia (*Tip 65*), such as abscesses, fistulae (seeping abscesses), and mastitis have been shown to occur much more frequently in smokers.

It is never too late to give up, and doing so will have immediate beneficial effects on your general health. It is especially important for women who are pregnant to stop smoking, because miscarriage, stillbirth, and premature or low-birthweight babies are more common in women who smoke.

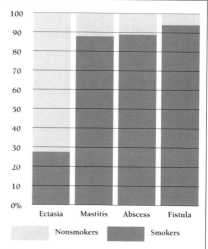

EFFECTS OF SMOKING
The percentage of women suffering from ectasia-related conditions is much higher in those who smoke than in the female population in general.

25 EXERCISE

Different types of exercise improve specific aspects of fitness. Aim to do aerobic exercise, such as swimming, and motor-fitness exercise, such as bike riding, as well as muscle toning and stretching.

MUSCLE TONING WITH FREE WEIGHTS
These two muscle-toning exercises using light weights will help improve your overall strength and fitness.

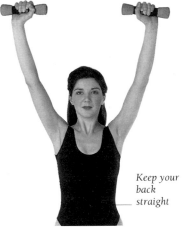

Keep your back straight

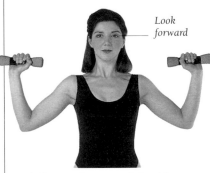

Look forward

1 △ To tone the arm and shoulder muscles, first bring your hands up to the height of your shoulders.

2 △ Keeping your back and head still, smoothly raise your arms above your head, then lower them. Repeat.

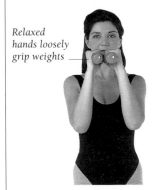

Relaxed hands loosely grip weights

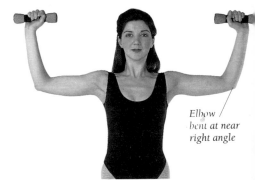

Elbow bent at near right angle

1 △ To tone your pectoral muscles, which can improve your cleavage, bring your hands together at chin level.

2 △ Gently move your hands out and apart, keeping them at chin level. Return to the start position, and repeat.

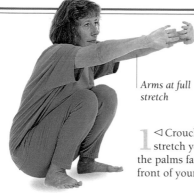

Arms at full stretch

STRETCHING
This exercise elongates the muscles and thus prevents muscle soreness, relaxes the body, and relieves tension. It is known as the good-morning stretch, and should be performed as one continuous movement.

Palms now facing forward

1 ◁ Crouch down and stretch your arms, with the palms facing outward, in front of your face.

Palms still facing out

2 ◁ Keeping your arms and hands outstretched, gradually straighten your legs and raise your buttocks.

Knees not locked

AEROBIC EXERCISE
Exercise in which muscles use up oxygen at the same rate as they receive it is called aerobic. Dancing, tennis, cycling, and fitness classes are all aerobic. You should do aerobic exercise nonstop for at least twenty minutes three times a week.

3 ▷ Rise up onto tiptoe, stretch your arms as high as you can above your head, and straighten your upper body. Slowly lower yourself back to the start position, and repeat.

Stretch toes and flex feet on tiptoe

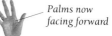

26 RELAXATION TECHNIQUES

You can reduce your stress levels, and so help to maintain good general health, by regularly practicing one or more relaxation techniques. These range from simple deep breathing exercises and relaxing of the muscles to more advanced techniques, such as yoga and meditation. Most relaxation methods are easily learned and practiced at home, but some (like yoga) need a teacher at first.

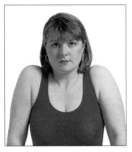

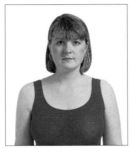

SHOULDER SHRUGS
Stress often results in pain and tension in the muscles of the neck and shoulders. Here is a simple exercise designed to relieve such tension. Take a deep breath as you tense your shoulders, and let it out when you relax them.

1 Tense your shoulder muscles by raising your shoulders as high as possible, and hold this position for a few seconds.

2 Allow the muscles to relax again by lowering your shoulders to their normal position. Repeat as necessary.

TENSE & RELAX ▽
Lie on your back, with knees bent and feet resting either on a chair or on the ground. Tense and relax each group of muscles in turn, from your feet up, inhaling as you tense and exhaling as you relax.

Begin the exercise at your feet

Breathe deeply and evenly

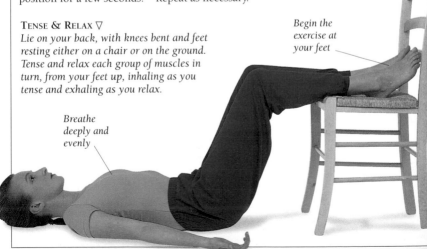

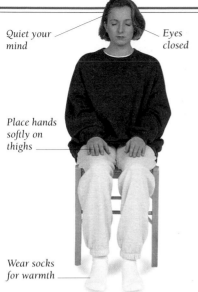

Quiet your mind

Eyes closed

Place hands softly on thighs

Wear socks for warmth

MEDITATION △
To promote physical well-being through mental relaxation, empty your mind of everyday thoughts and anxieties by focusing your attention on a word, phrase, or simple object.

YOGA ▽
Some types of yoga emphasize exercise, and others meditation. Both increase your suppleness and help quiet your mind through the practice of yoga postures and proper breathing. Look for a beginner's class with a sympathetic teacher.

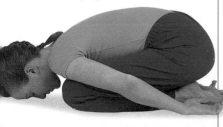

27 LIFE DECISIONS

How you make important decisions and cope with major life changes affects your overall health, and increases or reduces your risk of disease. Adopting a positive attitude toward life and change counters stress, and you can lower your chances of contracting breast cancer by doing the following:
- control your weight sensibly
- plan to have your first child before you reach the age of 30
- ideally, choose breast- rather than bottle-feeding (*Tip 39*)
- continue breast-feeding for as long as possible.

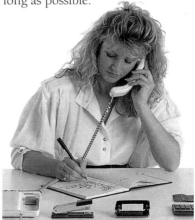

WORK & FAMILY
Many women now delay their first pregnancy until they are well into their 30s, because of work commitments and the need to build up financial reserves to support a family, but this delay can increase the risk of breast cancer.

THE SENSUAL BREAST

28 EROGENOUS ZONES

Certain areas of the body are particularly sensitive sexually; these are called erogenous zones. Women have more than men, perhaps because they are more important for female stimulation than visual or psychological stimuli. Erogenous zones may be stimulated by various kinds and intensities of touch.

TYPES OF EROGENOUS ZONE
Erogenous zones are classified, in order of sensitivity, as primary, secondary, or tertiary. A woman's primary zones are her external genital organs, and her lips, buttocks, and breasts.

NONPRIMARY ZONES
The ears, eyelids, cheeks, inner thighs, neck, and feet may also be sensitive areas, but these zones vary greatly from one individual to another.

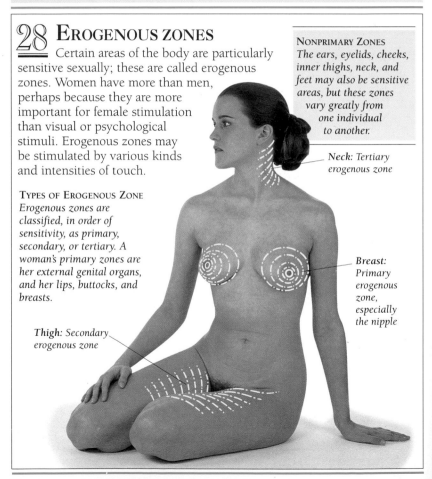

Neck: Tertiary erogenous zone

Breast: Primary erogenous zone, especially the nipple

Thigh: Secondary erogenous zone

29 NERVE SUPPLY

Sensory nerves carry signals such as touch, pain, and temperature. Each breast has an abundant supply, and these are responsible for the sensitivity of the areola and nipple.

Breasts also contain nerves from the autonomic nervous system, which controls involuntary body functions. These nerves probably make the connection between nipple stimulation and genital arousal and orgasm.

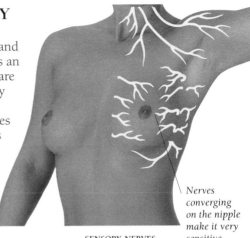

SENSORY NERVES

Nerves converging on the nipple make it very sensitive

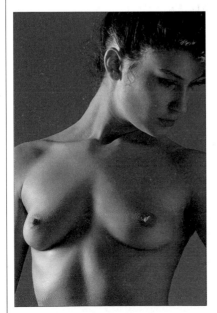

30 HOW BREASTS RESPOND

The breasts are one of a woman's primary erogenous zones, and they respond to direct stimulation during sexual arousal by becoming up to 25 percent larger. The nipples become erect, and the surrounding areolae darken.

In many women, dilated blood vessels and a consequent increased blood flow also cause a pink flush to extend over the front of the body, especially the chest. This is known as a sexual flush.

NIPPLE ERECTION
Small muscle fibers in the nipple contract, increasing both the length and diameter of the nipple. Even inverted nipples (Tip 65) respond a little to sexual stimulation.

31 EXPLORING YOUR BREASTS

To experience the pleasure that touching your own breasts can bring, try relaxing, breathing deeply, and exploring your breasts with your hands and fingers. Close your eyes and take your mind on a guided tour of each breast, concentrating on the variety of sensations.

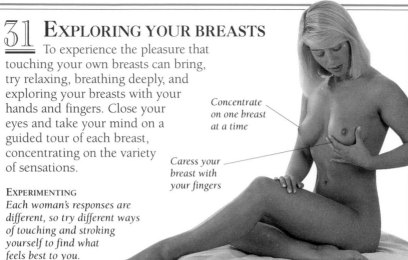

Concentrate on one breast at a time

Caress your breast with your fingers

EXPERIMENTING
Each woman's responses are different, so try different ways of touching and stroking yourself to find what feels best to you.

32 LEARN THROUGH SELF-STIMULATION

Many women enjoy the pleasures of masturbation, and arousing the breasts is an integral part of stimulating yourself. Start by caressing your breasts and, as they respond, increase the intensity of touch by squeezing, pressing, or running your fingernails over the nipple. This can increase sensations in other parts of your body.

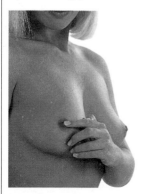

◁ **PRESSING**
Gently press on and around your nipples with your fingertip to stimulate and arouse them.

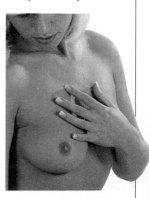

SQUEEZING ▷
Use the palm of your hand to squeeze and fondle each breast individually, noting how they both feel.

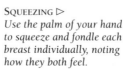

33 BREASTS IN FOREPLAY

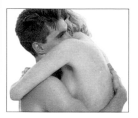

START WITH A HUG

During the prelude to intercourse with a partner, most women enjoy having their breasts touched in a variety of ways. Caressing with hands can lead to arousal, and the warm, wet feel of lips and tongue on your breasts, especially on the nipples, is usually very pleasurable – often to both partners.

34 STIMULATION BY YOUR PARTNER

Breast stimulation is also important just prior to and during intercourse itself. The "front to back" position makes it easy for your partner to reach around to fondle your breasts and nipples, and also to stimulate your clitoris if you wish.

REACHING ORGASM
For some women, nipple stimulation is essential in helping them achieve orgasm.

Swollen areola and erect nipple

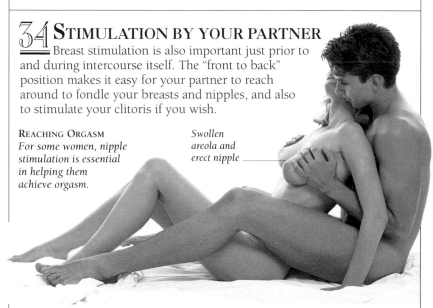

35 SEX & THE OLDER BREAST

Swelling of the breasts with sexual excitement becomes less and less as you age. This is because of the gradual loss of breast tissue and of elasticity in the tissue. By the age of 50, only about one-fifth of women experience an increase in breast size similar to when they were younger. Nipple erection still occurs, but often in only one breast. The sexual flush also appears much less frequently.

PREGNANCY & BREAST-FEEDING

36 MILK PRODUCTION (LACTATION)

During pregnancy, the milk glands and ducts begin to develop further as a result of the activity of several hormones. The cells lining the alveoli (milk-secreting glands) accumulate fat droplets and small granules of protein – the basic components of milk. These are released into alveolar sacs behind the nipple, and the breasts are fully capable of producing milk by the fifth or sixth month of pregnancy.

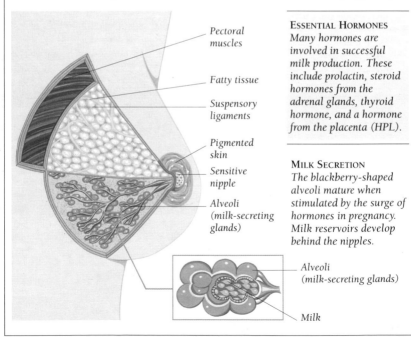

Pectoral muscles

Fatty tissue

Suspensory ligaments

Pigmented skin

Sensitive nipple

Alveoli (milk-secreting glands)

ESSENTIAL HORMONES
Many hormones are involved in successful milk production. These include prolactin, steroid hormones from the adrenal glands, thyroid hormone, and a hormone from the placenta (HPL).

MILK SECRETION
The blackberry-shaped alveoli mature when stimulated by the surge of hormones in pregnancy. Milk reservoirs develop behind the nipples.

Alveoli (milk-secreting glands)

Milk

37 CHANGES DURING PREGNANCY

Breast changes are one of the earliest signs of pregnancy and result from the secretion of the pregnancy hormone progesterone. Two of the first signs are swelling of the areola and rapid swelling of the breasts themselves.
- Most pregnant women experience tenderness in the breasts and nipples.
- Blood vessels become increasingly visible on the skin of the breasts.
- Nipples and areolae darken in color.

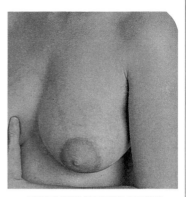

APPEARANCE CHANGES RAPIDLY

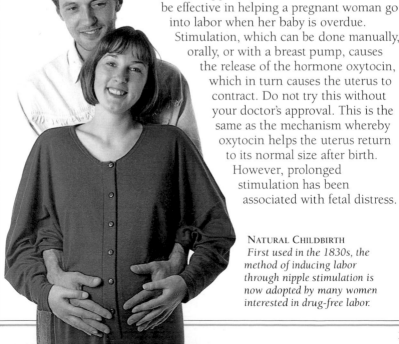

38 THE BREASTS & LABOR

Nipple stimulation has been found to be effective in helping a pregnant woman go into labor when her baby is overdue. Stimulation, which can be done manually, orally, or with a breast pump, causes the release of the hormone oxytocin, which in turn causes the uterus to contract. Do not try this without your doctor's approval. This is the same as the mechanism whereby oxytocin helps the uterus return to its normal size after birth. However, prolonged stimulation has been associated with fetal distress.

NATURAL CHILDBIRTH
First used in the 1830s, the method of inducing labor through nipple stimulation is now adopted by many women interested in drug-free labor.

39 WHY BREAST-FEED?

Every woman has the right to make her own choices at all stages of her life. Whether to feed your baby from the breast or from a bottle is a decision only you can make. There is a wealth of evidence, however, indicating that breast-feeding is better in a number of ways.

- Breast milk contains all the essential nutrients that a baby needs.
- Skin-to-skin contact gives your baby warmth and safety, and helps you both to bond.
- Many women enjoy breast-feeding.
- Breast-feeding can reduce your risk of developing breast cancer.

COLOSTRUM
A straw-colored fluid, known as colostrum, is produced by the breasts during late pregnancy and the first few days after birth. It has a high mineral and protein content, but is less fatty and sweet than breast milk. This makes it perfect for the baby's first food taken by mouth.

INVOLVING YOUR PARTNER
Make it a family experience by encouraging close physical contact between you, your partner, and your baby.

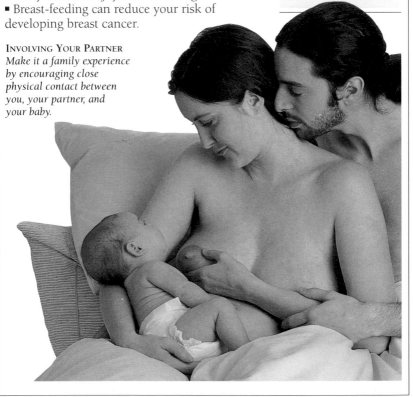

40 NUTRITION FOR NURSING MOTHERS

A nursing mother needs plenty of nutrients in her diet, as well as some extra calories. These should not be "empty" calories, from foods high in unnecessary fats and sugars but containing few other nutrients. The "extras" are best obtained from extra servings of meat or meat substitutes, fruit, vegetables, and breads.

PROTEIN
Cell-building protein is contained in sources such as meat, chicken, fish, beans, and tofu.

LENTILS

OILY FISH

VITAMIN A
Found in liver, leafy vegetables, and dairy products, vitamin A aids the immune system, the growth of bones and teeth, and cell development.

PARSLEY

FRUIT
Citrus and other fruits are an excellent source of additional calories, vitamins, and dietary fiber, and should be eaten in preference to candy and desserts.

CITRUS FRUIT

VITAMIN C
Most common in fruits and vegetables, this vitamin is essential to the production of collagen, the basis of bones, teeth, skin, and connective tissue.

RED PEPPER

VEGETABLES
These are packed with all the goodness of sun and soil, providing vitamins, minerals, and fiber. Eat plenty every day for health and energy.

BROCCOLI

VITAMIN E
Polyunsaturated oils, whole grains, nuts, and seeds provide this vitamin, which helps protect blood and lung cells from the harmful effects of oxidation.

PECANS

BREAD
Choose whole-grain breads and cereals, which have a much higher fiber and nutrient content than refined ones, but still provide carbohydrates.

WHOLE-GRAIN BREAD

ZINC
This mineral is found in meat, shellfish, peas, beans, yogurt, and whole-grain cereals. It promotes growth in children and boosts the immune system.

OATMEAL

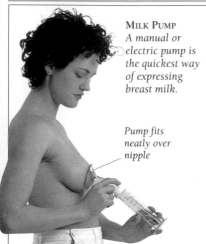

MILK PUMP
A manual or electric pump is the quickest way of expressing breast milk.

Pump fits neatly over nipple

41 EXPRESSING BREAST MILK

It may be convenient to express and freeze some of your breast milk. The best way of doing this is to use a pump, but you can hand-massage the breast. Expressing breast milk has several advantages.

- A partner or friend can feed your baby in your absence.
- It will relieve discomfort if your breasts have become too full.
- The baby can still receive breast milk if you are ill or too weak to breast-feed normally.

42 THE LET-DOWN REFLEX

The milk in a mother's breasts is not available for her baby until it has been let down (ejected) from the milk glands. For breast-feeding to go smoothly, regular let-down is essential. Let-down is stimulated by several factors, the strongest being the sensation of the baby sucking at the nipple. Some mothers' reflex occurs simply when the baby cries.

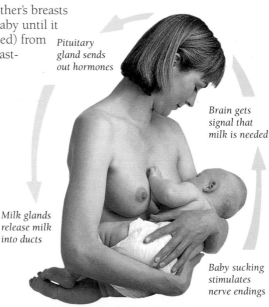

Pituitary gland sends out hormones

Brain gets signal that milk is needed

Milk glands release milk into ducts

Baby sucking stimulates nerve endings

MILK PRODUCTION
This is controlled by the hormones prolactin, which initiates milk production, and oxytocin, which forces milk into the ducts.

43 CAN YOU BREAST-FEED WHILE ILL?

If a breast-feeding mother becomes ill with a common cold or influenza, the only reason not to breast-feed is if she feels too ill to do so. Mother and baby will often be in close contact, so the baby is likely to pick up the infection anyway. A mother with a more serious illness can express milk (*Tip 41*) for her baby.

■ Breast-feeding can be beneficial to a diabetic mother, since it may reduce her need for insulin.
■ A cancerous breast lump poses no known risk to the baby. However, the mother will need immediate treatment. Avoiding breast-feeding is advisable if there is any question.
■ A mother who is HIV-positive should not breast-feed her baby.

44 BREAST-FEEDING PROBLEMS

It is natural for a woman to breast-feed her offspring, and her body is designed for this purpose, but problems may occur nevertheless. The most common of these are sore nipples, blocked ducts, engorgement, and breast abscess. Treatments are readily available, however, to alleviate the symptoms.

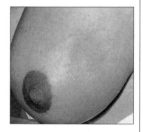

BREAST ABSCESS

HELP FOR COMMON CONDITIONS

Problem	Symptom(s)	Treatment
Sore nipples	Slightly tender, sore, or cracked nipples	Apply a special cream and use a nipple shield while breast-feeding
Blocked ducts	Tenderness and soreness of the breast, sometimes with reddening of the skin over the blockage	Feed your baby while massaging the breast above the sore area; if this fails, consult your doctor
Engorgement	Discomfort and feeling of fullness, tenderness, hardness, and pain	Express some milk from the breast to relieve it
Breast abscess	Swelling, tenderness, and reddening of an area of the breast	Your doctor will prescribe a course of antibiotics

CARING FOR YOUR BREASTS

45 BREAST EXERCISES

You can use exercise to strengthen and tone your pectoral muscles, but exercise won't actually change the shape or size of the breasts themselves. Toning the muscles may help lift the breasts and increase their bulk a little.

LEG PUSH-UPS
Perform this muscle-toning exercise several times with your right leg outstretched, and then repeat the whole sequence with your left leg.

WATCH YOUR BACK
You need to keep a straight back throughout the exercise, since arching it may cause damage.

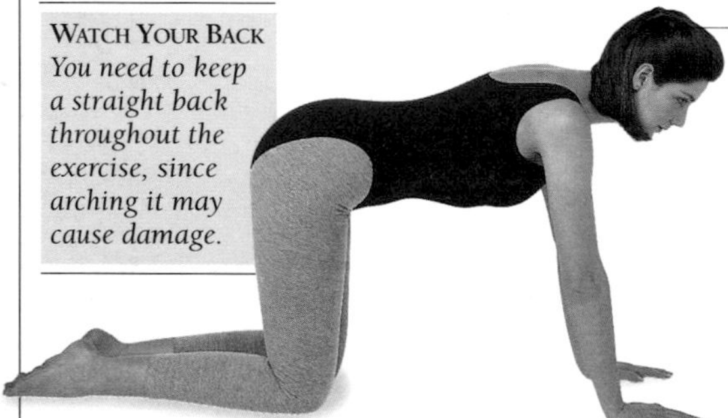

Keep head and neck relaxed

1 ◁ Kneel on all fours, with your hands shoulder-width apart, beneath your elbows. Keep your arms straight.

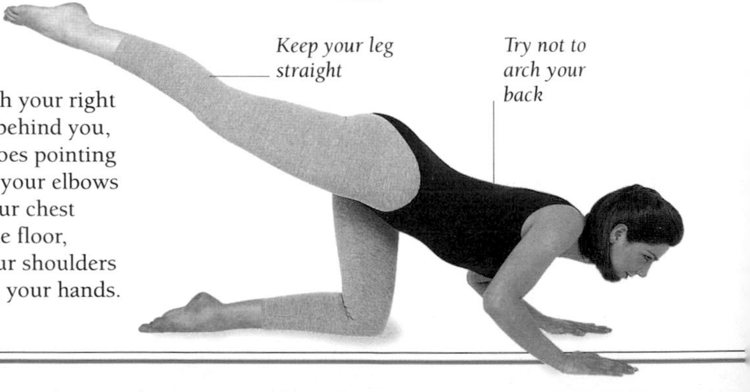

Keep your leg straight

Try not to arch your back

2 ▷ Stretch your right leg out behind you, with your toes pointing back. Bend your elbows to lower your chest nearly to the floor, keeping your shoulders in line with your hands.

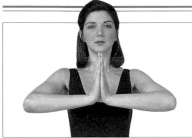

PALM PRESSES
Press your palms together in front of your breasts. Hold for five seconds, relax, and repeat the exercise ten times.

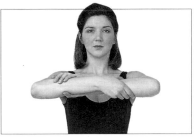

FOREARM GRIP
Grasp your forearms at shoulder level and then pull outward without letting go. Repeat the exercise ten times.

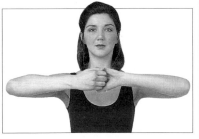

FINGER LOCK
Curl your fingers, lock them together at shoulder height, and pull. Hold for five seconds. Repeat the exercise ten times.

46 EVERYDAY CARE

The skin of the breasts is very delicate, and should be treated with care. "Beauty" treatments are generally worthless, however. Don't scrub or towel your breasts roughly, since this can make the nipples sore and tender.

If your nipples become dry and flaky just before your period, it's a good idea to moisturize them twice a week with a fragrance-free moisturizer. Any persistent patch of eczema (*Tip 67*) needs a doctor's attention.

SUN PROTECTION
Ideally, don't expose your skin to the sun for long periods. If you must do so, apply a sunblock with a protection factor greater than 15 every two hours or so.

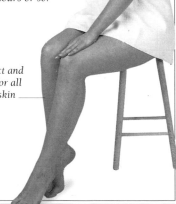
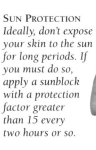
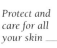

Protect and care for all your skin

47 EXAMINING YOUR BREASTS

Breast self-examination will help you to become familiar with your body. Ideally, it's best to start doing this when you are menstruating regularly and continue it throughout your life. For the first few months, examine your breasts at different times in the menstrual cycle so that you become familiar with changes in consistency. Then examine them once a month.

SELF-EXAMINATION: USING YOUR EYES
Do the same sequence of checks each month. Begin with a general visual examination, as shown here, then careful looking (Tip 48) and feeling (Tip 50).

1 ▷ In a warm place where you can be private, undress to the waist, and stand or sit in front of a mirror.

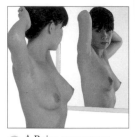

2 △ Raise your arms above your head and turn to each side to see your breasts in profile.

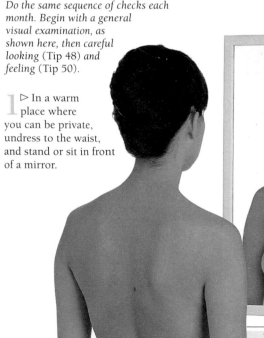

NORMAL LUMPINESS
Your breasts may normally become fuller and feel lumpy during the second half of your menstrual cycle.

48 SELF-EXAMINATION: LOOKING

Carefully study each breast in the mirror for changes in size, appearance, color of the nipples; differences in level between the nipples; eczema; or dimpling of the skin. Leaning forward can help highlight any changes that may not otherwise be obvious to you.

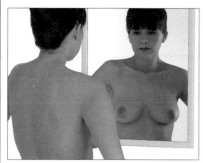

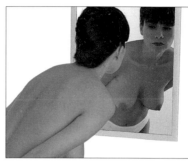

1 Place both your hands firmly on your hips and press them in hard. As you do this, you should feel your chest muscles beginning to tense.

2 Now lean forward. Look especially for dimpling or puckering of the skin, nipple retraction (when it appears pulled in), or a change in breast outline.

49 HOW YOUR PARTNER CAN HELP

Changes in a woman's breasts may be found first by her partner during lovemaking. If you're reluctant to touch your breasts, you may not be aware of anything unusual. Your partner can help by noting changes and discussing them unemotionally with you later.

LOVING ATTENTION
The sensitive touch of your partner can encourage you to become more familiar with your breasts.

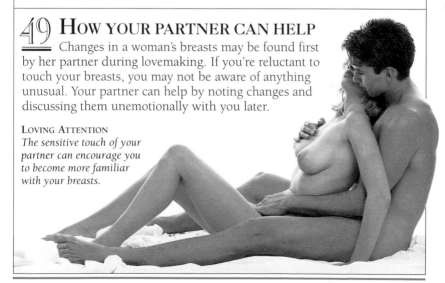

50 SELF-EXAMINATION: FEELING

After the visual examination, continue the process by feeling your breasts with your fingertips, keeping your fingers parallel to the skin of the breast. Using a soapy hand or a sprinkling of talcum powder helps the hand slide smoothly over the breast. Lying down with one arm behind your head shifts the breast tissue underneath your arm toward the center of your chest, giving you better access to it and making it easier for you to feel.

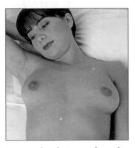

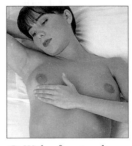

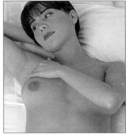

1 Lie back in a relaxed position and place your right arm behind your head. You may find that you need a pillow under your left shoulder.

2 With a firm touch, examine your right breast with your left hand, using any of the ways of feeling shown opposite (*Tip 51*).

3 Continue to check right into your armpit and along the top of your collarbone for lumps, which may be swollen lymph nodes.

4 Place your left hand behind your head and, using your right hand, examine your left breast and armpit in the same way.

Use the sensitive pads of your fingertips

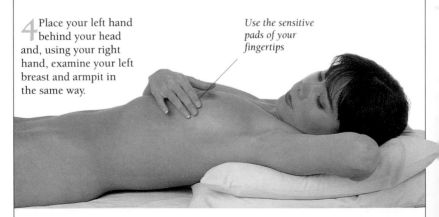

51 DIFFERENT WAYS OF FEELING

There are several different ways to feel the breasts during self-examination, and these are known as patterns of feeling, or palpation. Choose whichever is the most comfortable method for you, and take care to use the same pattern every time you examine yourself. A consistent approach will help you identify any changes early.

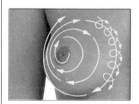

CONCENTRIC CIRCLES
Start with a large outer circle, making smaller circles with your fingers, and work your way in.

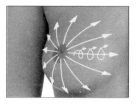

RADIAL PATTERN
Mentally divide the breast into a clock pattern. Work out toward 12 o'clock, then 1 o'clock, and so on.

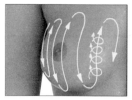

UP & DOWN
Imagine the breast as a series of vertical bands, and work your way up and down from the armpit.

52 NORMAL FINDINGS

Once you have examined your breasts a few times, you will know what is normal for you. You may find subtle changes such as tiny lumps, pronounced lumpiness, swelling of tissue between the nipple and the armpit or in the lower part of the breast, or scar tissue, which are all quite normal. From now on, though, you will be able to detect any major changes.

NATURAL CONDITIONS
When examining yourself, you may find things that cause you concern. Many of these, as shown here, are natural conditions and quite harmless.

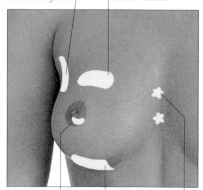

Bulge of tissue – the axillary tail

Pad of slightly thicker tissue

Hollow spot under nipple

Ridge of firm tissue under breast

Knobs where ribs and breastbone join

53 SIGNIFICANT CHANGES

Once you know what is normal for your breasts, be on the alert for any changes that will require a doctor's attention. While *looking* at your breasts, you may notice one or more of the following:

- Prominent veins
- Change of size in either breast
- New dimpling or puckering of skin
- Change in nipple appearance
- Nipple discharge or bleeding.

While *feeling* your breasts, you may find a new, distinct lump that fulfills the following criteria:

- It is obviously a lump, not just thickened breast tissue
- It remains unchanged throughout one or two menstrual cycles.

EXTRA ATTENTION
If you find a new lump in your breast, also examine your armpit and the top of your collarbone to see whether any of your lymph nodes are swollen as well.

NIPPLE DISCHARGE
Check for nipple discharge by examining your clothes. Don't squeeze the nipple, which can cause discharge where there was none. Discharge is significant only if it appears without squeezing, from one nipple only, or is persistent.

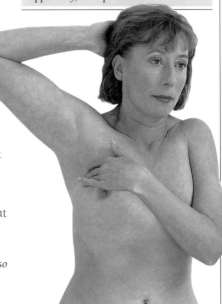

54 FINDING A LUMP

If you find a lump, but can't decide whether it is serious or not, consult your doctor anyway, if only to set your mind at ease. The vast majority of lumps detected through self-examination are not cancerous. On finding a lump, first check the same part of the other breast. If both your breasts feel the same, there is nothing to worry about. If one feels different from the other, arrange to see your gynecologist, who will refer you to a specialist for additional tests, if necessary. Moral support is especially valuable at this time.

55 TYPES OF LUMP

Only a proportion of breast lumps are cancerous. About 75 percent of all lumps are nonmalignant, and these include cysts (fluid-filled tissue sacs), fibroadenomas (tumors), and connective tissue hyperplasia (enlarged glands). Such forms of fibrocystic disease (benign breast tumors) affect about one-fifth of women between 20 and 50.

FREQUENCY OF CANCER DETECTION
The frequency with which cancer is detected in given parts of the breast is shown here in percentages.

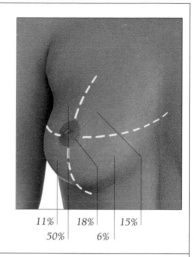

11% | 18% | 15%
50% | 6%

56 REGULAR SCREENING

Breast self-examination is recommended for all women, at all stages of their lives, but additional checks are advisable for older women, whose risk of breast cancer is higher, and for women in other high-risk groups (with breast cancer in the family, for example). Regular screening programs are advisable for women over 40, and should not be a cause for apprehension.

WHAT DOES IT INVOLVE?
The screening process consists of a physical examination by a doctor and a mammogram.

43

57 MAMMOGRAPHY

A mammogram is a low-dose X ray of the breast, designed to show the soft tissue very well. It is so refined that it can pick up small cancers and other abnormalities that can't be felt in a manual examination. The film is developed and examined by a radiologist who specializes in the interpretation of mammograms. The results take just a few days.

Mammograms are used for screening women over 40, since breast cancer is relatively rare in younger women and the density of their breasts makes the mammogram less effective. They are also used for women in high-risk categories.

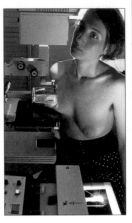

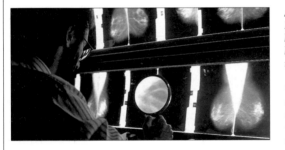

△ OBTAINING THE IMAGE
Each breast is compressed between two plates. If your breasts are painful, this may be uncomfortable.

◁ INTERPRETATION
An experienced radiologist scrutinizes the image on each mammogram for any sign of abnormality.

58 OTHER SCREENING TECHNIQUES

Mammography is the most widely used method of imaging the breast, but there are some other techniques that you may come across, especially if you are referred for additional tests after a routine screening mammogram.

- Xero-mammography requires different equipment than normal mammography, and gives an end product on paper rather than film.

- Ultrasound produces a picture similar to an X-ray photograph. Patterns are produced by echoes of sound waves bouncing off tissue. Ultrasound is good for examining dense breasts, and is painless.
- Thermography works by mapping out tissue temperatures using infrared photography.
- Other new techniques are constantly being developed.

BENIGN BREAST CHANGES

59 WHAT CAUSES BREAST PAIN?

Many women suffer from breast pain (mastalgia), and may fear that cancer is the cause. In fact, noncyclical pain (pain not linked to the menstrual cycle) that seems to be in the breast may be musculoskeletal and originate from some other part of the body. Cyclical breast pain is usually linked to menstruation.

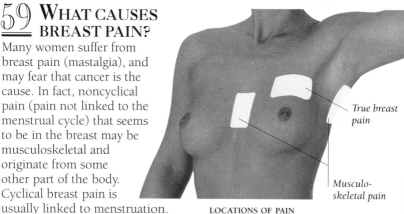

True breast pain

Musculo-skeletal pain

LOCATIONS OF PAIN

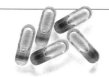

EVENING PRIMROSE CAPSULES

ALLEVIATING THE PAIN
Evening primrose oil is effective, but it must be taken in a large dose over several months before showing really positive results.

EVENING PRIMROSE FLOWER

60 CYCLICAL BREAST PAIN

The most common kind of true breast pain is associated with the menstrual cycle. Most women experience some degree of breast pain when their breasts become sensitive just prior to menstruation. Some, however, may experience soreness and tenderness for about two weeks from the middle of the cycle until menstruation takes place. Treatments include evening primrose oil (avoid in pregnancy) and certain prescription drugs. Consult your doctor.

45

61 NONCYCLICAL BREAST PAIN

There are two types of noncyclical breast pain: true breast pain, which comes from the breast but is unrelated to the menstrual cycle, and pain felt in the region of the breast but actually coming from somewhere else. The latter is known as musculoskeletal pain.

- True breast pain is sometimes associated with benign breast conditions, such as duct ectasia.
- Pain in the breasts may originate in the chest wall or spine, and is often caused by a kind of arthritis.
- If your pain occurs in one spot only, and is constant, see a doctor.

62 BENIGN LUMPS

Every woman has a lump – or general lumpiness – somewhere in her breasts, and the most common breast lumps belong to a group of harmless conditions that are merely a variation of normal. There are only two kinds of benign breast lump; these are called fibroadenomas and cysts.

▽ LOCATION OF LUMPS
If you find a lump, your doctor will give you a physical examination and note the location of the lump. He or she will also examine the armpit for swollen lymph nodes.

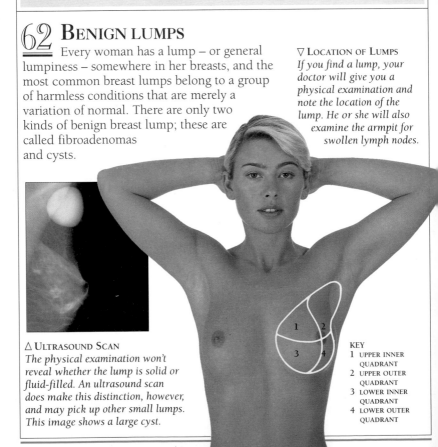

△ ULTRASOUND SCAN
The physical examination won't reveal whether the lump is solid or fluid-filled. An ultrasound scan does make this distinction, however, and may pick up other small lumps. This image shows a large cyst.

KEY
1 UPPER INNER QUADRANT
2 UPPER OUTER QUADRANT
3 LOWER INNER QUADRANT
4 LOWER OUTER QUADRANT

63 FIBROADENOMAS

These completely benign lumps are common in teenagers and women in their 20s, and are simply over-developed lobules. They can be any size from a pea to a lemon, and are often found near the nipple. They feel smooth, firm, and distinct, and move freely in the breast. Such a lump need not be removed, since most will shrink.

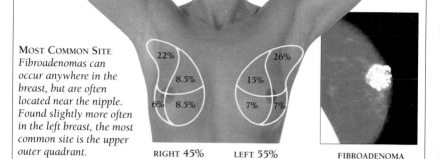

MOST COMMON SITE
Fibroadenomas can occur anywhere in the breast, but are often located near the nipple. Found slightly more often in the left breast, the most common site is the upper outer quadrant.

RIGHT 45%   LEFT 55%

FIBROADENOMA

64 ARE CYSTS A DISEASE?

Cysts are fluid-filled sacs, caused by the blockage of glands as they change through life. As such, cysts are just a variation of normal breast anatomy, and not a disease.

Cysts may appear suddenly, and are common in women in their 30s, 40s, and 50s. Your doctor will use fine-needle aspiration cytology (FNAC) to confirm the diagnosis.

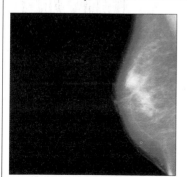

CYST MAMMOGRAM
Mammography will detect a cyst, but cannot distinguish between it and other breast lumps. Here, the cyst appears as an irregular white area behind the nipple.

TREATMENT IS PAINLESS
FNAC serves as both diagnosis and treatment in one. Aspiration is a simple, quick, and painless procedure. All you will feel is a needle prick, as the fluid is drawn into a syringe. The cyst collapses and disappears.

65 ECTASIA & RELATED NIPPLE DISORDERS

Benign changes to the nipple are less common than other breast disorders, but can be equally troubling and should be promptly assessed by a doctor. The normal shrinkage of milk ducts in a woman's 40s and 50s can lead to nipple disorders. Dilation of the ducts (ectasia) may lead to various problems (*below*).

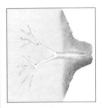

In normal ectasia, the ducts become dilated and fluid stagnates.

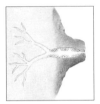

The lining of the ducts may become ulcerated and cause a discharge.

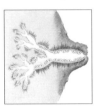

Fluid may leak into surrounding tissue, causing painful swelling.

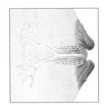

Scarred, shrinking tissue may pull the nipple in, causing it to become inverted.

66 NIPPLE DISCHARGE

Most instances of nipple discharge have a benign cause and are best left alone, but if the discharge is profuse, bloodstained, or persistent, consult your doctor, who will perform a biopsy. There may be needle-shaped deposits of calcium in the milk ducts or an ulcerated duct. Seriously affected ducts can be surgically removed.

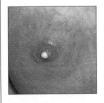

MILKY DISCHARGE
Breasts sometimes secrete milk in a woman who is not breast-feeding, a condition known as galactorrhea.

67 SKIN CONDITIONS

Cracked nipples during breast-feeding may be a problem (*Tip 44*). Don't confuse eczema, an easily treatable condition, with Paget's disease, a form of cancer. If in any doubt, consult your doctor.

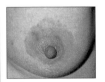

ECZEMA
Recurrent scaly, red, itchy patches around the nipple usually respond to hydrocortisone cream treatment.

PAGET'S DISEASE
This is actually a slow-growing form of breast cancer, but it is easily confused with eczema.

BREAST CANCER

68 HOW COMMON IS BREAST CANCER?

In the US, breast cancer affects around one in every ten women over a lifetime, which in real terms means one in 1,000 of the women living around you at any one time. Five times more women suffer from the disease than die from it. With each year you live without developing breast cancer, your chances of dying from it decrease. In statistical terms, it is the leading female cancer, and the most common cause of death in women between 35 and 55. Beyond this age, heart disease kills many more women.

MALIGNANCY
For every cancerous breast lump found, ten others are harmless. Even with cancerous lumps, 8 out of 10 women survive for at least five years.

FATAL DISEASES
In the US among women of all ages, cardiovascular disease and stroke cause many more deaths than breast cancer.

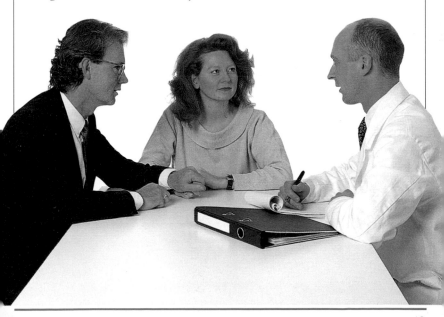

69 RISK FACTORS & PROTECTION

Some women are more likely to get breast cancer than others, because of genetic or environmental factors, and sometimes a combination of the two. Risk factors include:

- a family history of breast cancer
- a high level of female hormones
- the early onset and late cessation of menstruation
- having your first child after the age of 30, or remaining childless.

The best protection against breast cancer is pregnancy, the earlier the better, followed by breast-feeding.

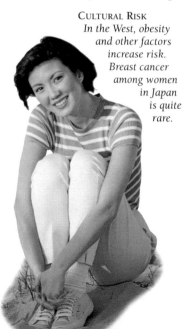

CULTURAL RISK
In the West, obesity and other factors increase risk. Breast cancer among women in Japan is quite rare.

70 HEREDITARY BREAST CANCER

A family history of breast cancer is a strong risk factor in itself, and it also makes all other risk factors potentially more dangerous. The increase in risk depends on how close the relative is, and on how many relatives have had breast cancer. A woman whose mother developed cancer in both breasts before the age of 35, for example, has a 50 percent chance of developing breast cancer herself.

RISK FACTOR	
25 times normal risk	MOTHER WITH BILATERAL BREAST CANCER UNDER 35
20 times normal risk	MOTHER & SISTER WITH BREAST CANCER
15 times normal risk	SISTER WITH BILATERAL BREAST CANCER UNDER 40
10 times normal risk	SISTER WITH BILATERAL BREAST CANCER UNDER 50
5 times normal risk	FIRST-DEGREE RELATIVE (MOTHER OR SISTER) WITH BREAST CANCER
normal risk	SECOND-DEGREE RELATIVE (AUNT OR GRANDMOTHER) WITH BREAST CANCER

HOW HEREDITARY FACTORS INCREASE RISK

71 PREVENTIVE MEASURES

There are some factors you can control to reduce your risk of breast cancer. Eating a balanced diet, restricting alcohol intake to moderate levels, having an early first child, and breast- rather than bottle-feeding will all lower your risk. For women at very high risk, however, some other kind of prevention may be advisable.

■ Tamoxifen is a complex hormonal drug that is used in the treatment of women who already have cancer in one breast (*Tip 86*). In the long term, it reduces by half the risk of getting cancer in the other breast.
■ Prophylactic (preventive) mastectomy may very occasionally be advisable in the case of women with an extremely high risk level.

72 THE NATURE OF BREAST CANCER

Breast cancer is not a single entity, but a family of conditions. The common feature of every type, however, is that certain cells start to grow out of control. This abnormal cell growth is rapid, and absorbs a great deal of body energy. In the breast, where tissue is solid, the fast-growing cancer cells produce a swelling, or tumor. Most tumors are not malignant, don't spread, and are not fatal. Malignant tumors, however, are invasive, and spread beyond their original location, either into surrounding fat, muscles, or skin, or through the blood or lymphatic fluid to other organs of the body.

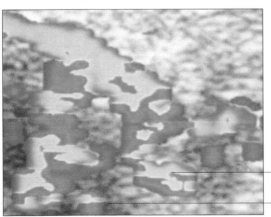

ULTRASOUND IMAGE
Color can be added to an ultrasound image to show the rate of blood flow. The colored areas represent an increased flow rate. Although a rich blood supply to a tumor is a strong clue to malignancy, it would not on its own be a basis for firm diagnosis.

Colored areas represent increased blood flow

Cancer shows up as a shadowed area

73 NONINVASIVE CANCER

Overgrowth of cells may occur throughout a woman's fertile life in any part of the lobes or ducts in her breasts. This is called hyperplasia and is a benign condition. In some hyperplasias, however, the cells become atypical, and may turn into a localized cancer. Noninvasive cancer in situ carries a high risk of becoming invasive.

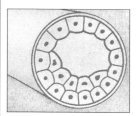

1 In hyperplasia, the cells in the duct multiply more than is necessary, creating a harmless excess that builds up inside the duct.

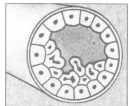

2 In atypical hyperplasia, the cells lose their normal appearance, and are called "atypical." This is still a benign condition.

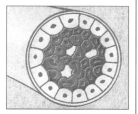

3 In cancer in situ, the atypical cells fill up the duct, forming a malignant carcinoma. At this stage they are still not invasive.

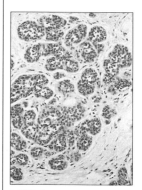

LCIS CELLS
Cells are uniform, small, and round. The glands can be seen, but are abnormal because they are not hollow. The nuclei are dark.

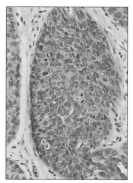

DCIS CELLS
A single gland is visible here, in which the cells are not uniform, have no recognizable structure, and are filling the space.

◁ **IN SITU CANCERS**
There are two kinds: ductal carcinoma in situ (DCIS) and lobular carcinoma in situ (LCIS). The words in situ are Latin for "in its place of origin."

PREINVASIVE DISEASE
LCIS in itself does not develop into cancer, but shows that a woman is at risk for developing DCIS, the extreme end of hyperplasia. DCIS is usually either focal (in one spot only) or multicentric (in several places).

74 TRUE CANCER

Breast cancers usually arise from the cells that line the ducts or lobules. The most frequent form is called ductal carcinoma, because at first it was thought to arise from the milk ducts. It is now known that this – and the less common lobular carcinoma – usually arise in the lobule. Both can be preinvasive (*Tip 73*) or invasive.

■ Invasive ductal carcinomas comprise over 80 percent of all detected breast cancers. The first symptom is generally a new, hard, ill-defined lump within the breast. As the tumor spreads along the ligaments between the breast lobes, it pulls on the overlying skin, creating a dimpling effect. The nipple may become inverted, and the lymph nodes may also be affected.

■ Invasive lobular carcinomas account for about 10 percent of breast cancers. They behave in a similar way to ductal cancers, but may spread diffusely rather than forming a discrete tumor.

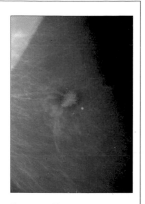

INVASIVE TUMOR
The area colored red in the center of this mammogram is a true cancer. The uneven "starburst" outline is typical of an invasive tumor.

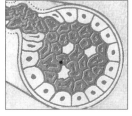

INVASIVE CARCINOMA
Once the cells begin to break out of the duct or lobule in which they originated, and spread out into the surrounding tissue, the cancer becomes truly invasive. At this stage of the disease, some form of surgery will almost always be required.

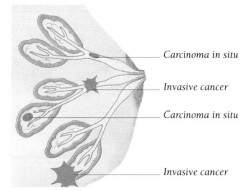

Carcinoma in situ

Invasive cancer

Carcinoma in situ

Invasive cancer

SITES OF CANCER
Breast cancer can arise in either the lobules or, more rarely, the milk ducts. If it remains confined to the lobule or duct, it is termed a carcinoma in situ. Once it spreads to the surrounding tissue, it is a true invasive cancer.

75 DETECTION & DIAGNOSIS

Doctors have many different investigative techniques and skills at their disposal in order to reach as specific a diagnosis as possible when a woman finds a lump in her breast. The first examination is a physical one, along the lines of your own self-examination. Then, in all cases, a sample of either cells or tissue is examined under a microscope to determine whether the lump is malignant. If it is, further tests are carried out to assess the precise origin of the tumor, its grade, and stage of development (*Tip 76*). Any discharge from the nipple is also tested.

SEQUENCE OF TESTS
So that you can be given the best treatment available, a number of tests are carried out on a lump to determine whether you have cancer and, if so, what type it is.

Referral to a Specialist
If something unusual shows up on a routine screening mammogram, or you find a lump during self-examination and notify your doctor, you may be referred to a specialist. First tests depend on whether there is a high probability of cancer.

Cancer Unlikely
Fine-needle aspiration cytology (FNAC) is used to analyze a sample of cells.

Cancer Possible
If cancer is suspected, revealed in FNAC, or FNAC is inconclusive, a biopsy will be required.

Biopsy
A cutting-needle or open biopsy is carried out to provide a sample of tissue from the lump.

Histology
Analysis of tissue slices (histology) diagnoses the cancer type and grades the tumor.

Further Tests
These will determine whether the cancer has spread, and will help in planning treatment.

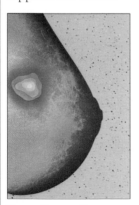

TUMOR DEEP IN BREAST
The yellow core in this enhanced mammogram indicates a cancerous tumor deep in the breast.

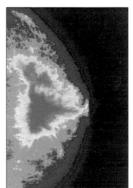
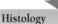

TUMOR IN MILK DUCT
The red area indicates a large malignant tumor in the mammary duct, containing dense tissue.

76 HOW FAR HAS IT PROGRESSED?

Your doctor will use a series of tests to discover the grade of the tumor (how aggressive it is), the stage of the disease (how far advanced it is), and whether it has spread. Once these factors have been determined, your doctor will be able to decide on the best form of treatment for your cancer, and assess your long-term outlook.

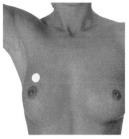

△ STAGE I
The disease is confined to the breast, with or without dimpling of the skin.

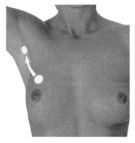

△ STAGE II
The axillary lymph nodes are affected. Stages I and II may be curable by surgery alone, but systemic treatment such as chemotherapy may also be advised.

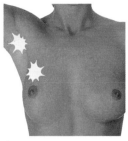

△ STAGE III
The cancer has invaded the muscles of the chest wall, the overlying skin, or possibly even the lymph nodes situated above the collarbone.

◁ STAGE IV
The cancer has spread to several other parts of the body. Typical sites for such secondary spread are the bones, liver, and lungs. The prognosis at this stage of development would be poor.

Lungs

Liver

Bones

PROGNOSIS & OUTLOOK
It is always difficult to give a precise outlook. Statistics show, however, that the five-year survival rate of 85 percent for Stage I tumors falls to less than 10 percent for Stage IV.

TREATING CANCER

77 BREAST CONSERVATION

The current approach is to conserve as much of the breast as possible by performing the least amount of surgery necessary. If your lump is less than 1½in (4cm) in diameter, it is suitable for treatment such as lumpectomy.

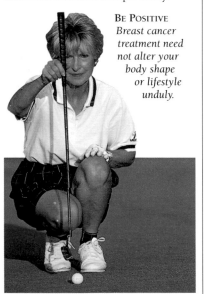

BE POSITIVE
Breast cancer treatment need not alter your body shape or lifestyle unduly.

78 TREATMENT OPTIONS

If you are diagnosed as having breast cancer, you should be fully aware of the treatment options open to you. Advanced techniques mean that you can be placed in a clearly defined group, and given a tailor-made treatment program.

- Lumpectomy (*Tip 79*) removes the lump, leaving the breast intact.
- Partial mastectomy (*Tip 80*) removes part of the breast.
- Total (or simple) mastectomy (*Tip 81*) removes all of the breast tissue.
- Modified radical mastectomy (*Tip 82*) removes all breast tissue and the muscle behind the breast.
- Radiation, chemotherapy, or hormones may be used after surgery.

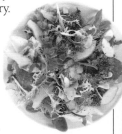

LIGHT FOOD
Chemotherapy (Tip 85) *may make you feel sick. Try eating light meals only, or ask your doctor or nurse for advice.*

79 LUMPECTOMY

This is now the preferred choice of treatment for breast cancer, wherever possible, because of its efficacy, its cosmetic qualities, and the fact that it is emotionally less traumatic. The operation is fairly minor, and is carried out under general anesthetic. You may have to stay in the hospital for four to five days to make sure the scar is healing and there are no complications.

EXTENT OF SURGERY
Your surgeon will remove the lump, with probably ½in (1cm) of healthy tissue around it, and the lymph nodes in the armpit.

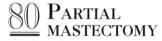

Lymph nodes usually removed as a precaution

80 PARTIAL MASTECTOMY

Where the cancer has no distinct outline, your surgeon will remove it together with a larger amount of surrounding tissue. Segmental excision and quadrantectomy are versions of partial mastectomy, and remove varying amounts of tissue. The operation can leave a misshapen breast, depending on how much tissue is removed. Knowing this, some women opt for a total mastectomy (*Tip 81*).

EXTENT OF SURGERY
A larger amount of the tissue surrounding the lump is removed than for a lumpectomy, and the lymph nodes are either sampled or removed.

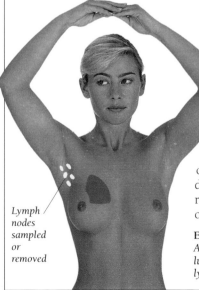

Lymph nodes sampled or removed

81 TOTAL (OR SIMPLE) MASTECTOMY

Mastectomy is a major operation involving removal of the entire breast; expect to stay in the hospital for up to eight days, depending on the extent of the surgery performed. If your shoulder is stiff afterward, there are some gentle exercises (*Tip 89*) that will help you get it back to normal.

EXTENT OF SURGERY
All of the breast tissue is removed, including the nipple and areola, the axillary tail that extends into the armpit, and some axillary nodes.

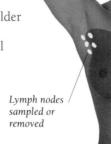

Lymph nodes sampled or removed

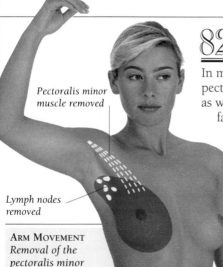

Pectoralis minor muscle removed

Lymph nodes removed

ARM MOVEMENT
Removal of the pectoralis minor muscle may result in restricted arm movement.

82 MODIFIED RADICAL MASTECTOMY

In modified radical mastectomy, the pectoralis minor muscle is removed as well as the breast tissue, to facilitate full axillary clearance. True radical mastectomy, in which the pectoralis major muscle is also removed, is no longer performed, so don't agree to it; insist upon getting a second opinion.

EXTENT OF SURGERY
Your surgeon will remove all of the breast tissue and the pectoralis minor muscle behind the breast, plus the axillary nodes.

83 TREATING AXILLARY DISEASE

When a lymph node has been infiltrated by cancer, it ceases to perform any useful service to your body, and cancer can only spread further. Therefore, affected axillary nodes must be removed or treated aggressively with radiation.

There is some debate as to the best treatment, but most specialists agree that complete removal should be the first step. Surgery enables sampling of the nodes as well as removal, and this helps in determining the stage of the disease. The nodes are classified into Levels I, II, and III, according to how deep they lie.

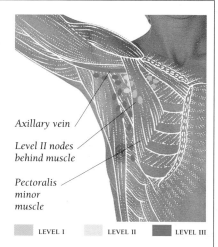

Axillary vein

Level II nodes behind muscle

Pectoralis minor muscle

▨ LEVEL I   ▨ LEVEL II   ▨ LEVEL III

STAGING THE AXILLA
When there is no Level I involvement in the cancer, the likelihood of disease at Levels II and III is very slight.

84 RADIATION

Some specialists advocate the use of radiation alone for treatment of axillary disease. Its normal application, however, is as an additional (adjuvant) treatment after surgery has been performed.

Doses of high-energy X rays are accurately beamed at the breast area of the chest wall to make sure that any remaining cancer cells are destroyed. This treatment is quite safe and should cause no alarm.

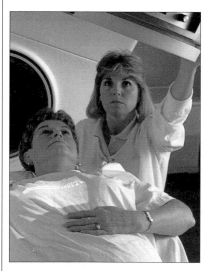

RADIATION SESSION
The radiologist asks you to raise one arm, sets up the machine, then leaves the room during the actual treatment.

85 CHEMOTHERAPY

For premenopausal women, chemotherapy, in which cytotoxic drugs find and kill cancer cells anywhere in the body, is often used after breast-cancer surgery. In some cases, chemotherapy is used as a preoperative measure, or may be the only treatment.

Treatment is usually given in cycles at monthly intervals by injection or drip. Side effects can be a problem. These include damage to bone marrow, tiredness, nausea, hair loss, mouth ulcers, loss of appetite, and diarrhea. Ask for advice on dealing with these.

86 HORMONE TREATMENT

Breast cancers are sometimes influenced by hormones, and lowering estrogen levels in the body may help combat cancer.
▪ For postmenopausal women, the anti-estrogen drug tamoxifen (*Tip 71*) is often effective after surgery. It has few side effects.
▪ For premenopausal women, removal of the ovaries (ablation) by surgery or radiation abolishes the secretion of estrogen.
▪ The injection of goserelin inhibits the brain hormones that control the ovaries' output of estrogen.

87 BREAST RECONSTRUCTION

If you have lost part or all of your breast, you should seriously consider reconstructive surgery, no matter what your long-term outlook may be. If your doctor is reluctant to explore the option, seek a second opinion. Your breast will be refashioned using either an implant or your own fat and muscle by way of a "flap" operation, of which there are several variations. Make sure you discuss all your options with your doctor before proceeding.

Expander implants are usually a first step to a permanent implant. Increasing amounts of fluid are injected into the expander bag over a period of time until enough space has been created for the permanent implant to be inserted.

RECTUS ABDOMINUS FLAP
A flap is taken from the rectus abdominus muscle with its blood supply, and repositioned. The new breast mound is stitched.

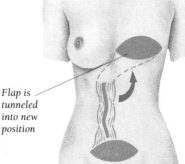

Flap is tunneled into new position

LIFE AFTER TREATMENT

88 ADJUSTING TO YOUR NEW BODY

All your medical caregivers are aware of the difficult adjustments to be made when treatment is complete and will give you counseling and support. Losing a breast is emotionally traumatic and getting used to your new shape takes time. You may opt for a breast prosthesis and will need to become comfortable with it. Exercises to strengthen your arm muscles will probably be routine.

LYMPHEDEMA
Painful swelling of the arm, which is caused by surgery on the axilla or radical radiation, arises very occasionally. Protect your arm, and raise it whenever possible.

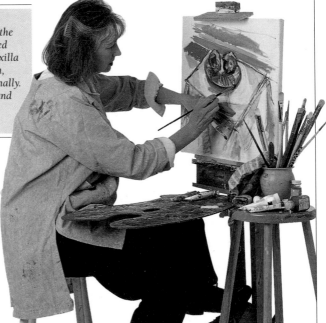

CONFIDENCE
Once treatment is over, you can start to regain your confidence, for example, by rediscovering favorite hobbies and pastimes.

89 POSTMASTECTOMY EXERCISES

Immediately after your operation, you may find that your shoulder movement is restricted.

Here are a few simple exercises that will help restore normal movement and flexibility.

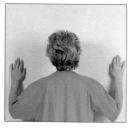

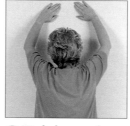

◁ **WALL REACHING**
Stand facing a wall with your feet apart, and work your hands up and down the wall. Don't lean your weight on your arms, and stop if you begin to feel any discomfort.

1 Place the palms of your hands flat against the wall at about shoulder or neck height.

2 Work them up the wall, then slide them down, and repeat. Try to reach higher each time.

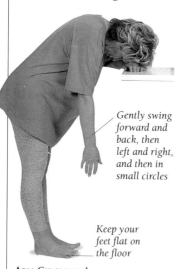

Straighten one arm at a time

Gently swing forward and back, then left and right, and then in small circles

Keep your feet flat on the floor

ARM CIRCLING △
Rest your good arm and your head on a flat surface, and swing your affected arm.

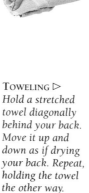

TOWELING ▷
Hold a stretched towel diagonally behind your back. Move it up and down as if drying your back. Repeat, holding the towel the other way.

90 BREAST PROSTHESES

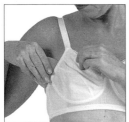

A prosthesis is a false breast put in a bra. It has no nipple and resembles the texture, fullness, and shape of a real breast. Lightweight, temporary prostheses are used as soon as your scar is healed, and later you will be fitted with a permanent, heavy one that "gives" to the touch and feels much like a normal breast.

USING A PROSTHESIS
Slip it into the special pocket inside your bra, to fill the cup.

△ BUST CUP   △ LIGHTWEIGHT
PROSTHESIS

△ TEARDROP SHAPE

△ UNDERARM EXTENSION

◁ PUSH-UP PAD

BRA FILLERS
Push-up pads and bust cups are available to fill out your bra after partial mastectomy.

△ TINTED

△ TRIANGULAR

SILICONE PROSTHESES
Permanent breast prostheses are made from silicone, a material that is soft to the touch but simulates the weight and droop of a normal breast. There are different types and shapes to suit your particular needs. Silicone nipples are available; these adhere to the prosthesis when moistened, making the breast more realistic.

△ NIPPLES

91 RECURRENCE & RISK

If you have survived breast cancer, you will still be concerned about follow-up treatment and the risk of any recurrence. The longer you live cancer free, the higher are your chances of a complete cure. Most doctors believe you should be carefully monitored for at least five years to detect possible recurrences or secondary spread of the disease.

- Survival for ten years or longer without recurrence or spread could indicate that you are cured.
- Local recurrence in the treated area can be cured by radiation or additional surgery.
- Recurrence in the scar or chest wall or in your other breast, or a new cancer in another part of your body all need urgent attention.

COSMETIC SURGERY

92 WHY HAVE SURGERY?

The importance of a woman's breasts to her self-image is – rightly or wrongly – reinforced by media images. This has led to a growing acceptance of every woman's right to alter her breasts with cosmetic surgery.

It is vital, however, that you have the operation for the correct reasons, and not because others are critical of your figure. You will never be happy with the results if this is the case. Be sure that *you* are making the decisions.

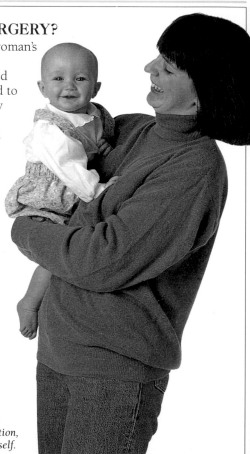

LOOK BEFORE YOU LEAP
Many women think that having cosmetic surgery on their breasts will dramatically change their lives. This very rarely turns out to be true, so think very carefully before going ahead.

LOOKING YOUNGER
One good reason for having plastic surgery is that your body may look older than you feel. After the operation, you may be more at ease with yourself.

93 CHOOSING A SURGEON

Women have undergone breast surgery for almost 100 years, and plastic surgeons have a great deal of experience. It is vital to find a good surgeon with whom you can establish an easy rapport.

- Get a reliable recommendation, preferably from your own doctor or a friend who has had cosmetic surgery.
- Don't rely on a newspaper or magazine advertisement.
- A good surgeon will advise you on the best procedure.
- An honest surgeon will never guarantee 100 percent success.

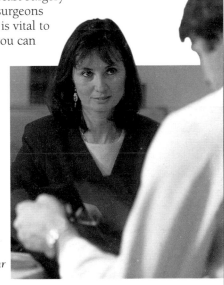

ESTABLISHING A RAPPORT
Entrust yourself to a surgeon only if you strike up a good relationship from the start. If you don't like the surgeon at your first visit, you're unlikely to later on.

94 PREPARING YOURSELF FOR SURGERY

Before going ahead with the operation, you should take time to weigh all the advantages and disadvantages that are associated with cosmetic breast surgery. Bear the following points in mind:

- Surgery can be very expensive
- Results may not be as good as you expect, or complications may arise
- You will suffer some discomfort, and possibly some scarring
- All surgery has a degree of risk.

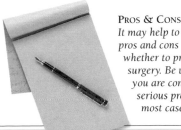

SCARRING
A good surgeon will hide scars in natural skin lines. Occasionally, however, they remain visible. Ask your surgeon what the extent will be.

PROS & CONS
It may help to make a list of pros and cons when deciding whether to proceed with surgery. Be under no illusions: you are contemplating a serious procedure that is in most cases unnecessary.

95 QUESTIONS TO ASK YOUR PLASTIC SURGEON

Cosmetic surgery involves a two-way contract between you and your surgeon. He or she owes you the best treatment, but you need to have thought out your decision in some detail, and have a realistic view of what the procedure and the results will be like. Here are questions to consider asking your surgeon before going ahead with any form of cosmetic surgery.

- Are there any preconditions necessary for this type of surgery?

- What are the general risks associated with surgery (especially for an older woman)?
- How likely is it that the results will not turn out as planned?
- Is it possible that complications could delay my recovery?
- How sore or painful will it be just after the operation, and for how long will this discomfort last?
- How visible or extensive will the scars from the surgery be, and will they ever disappear completely?

96 CORRECTING INVERTED NIPPLES

Breasts and nipples vary greatly from woman to woman, but one of the most common variations is inverted nipples (*Tip 65*). These can frequently be everted (turned out) simply by wearing breast "shells" over a period of a few weeks.

If this does not work, it may be that your nipples are held down by straps of fine tissue, usually caused by short ducts (a condition present from birth). This can easily be corrected by surgery (under local anesthetic), requiring only a few hours in the hospital. The straps of fine tissue are cut to release the nipple.

AFTEREFFECTS OF SURGERY
You'll soon be back on your feet, but you won't know for certain whether you can breast-feed until your breasts become active during pregnancy.

97 BREAST REDUCTION

Women who have very large breasts sometimes dislike them because they are heavy or feel socially embarrassing. Others wish to have firm, well-positioned breasts. Both these situations can be improved with a breast reduction operation. Your surgeon will advise what size and shape your breasts should be after surgery.

Skin and tissue to be removed

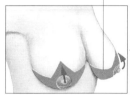

Nipple and areola under the skin

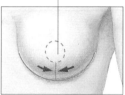

Nipple and areola in new position

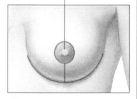

1 △ Tissue is removed, and the nipple and areola are moved up on a pedicle (stalk of tissue).

2 △ The skin edges are stitched together, leaving the nipple and areola temporarily inside.

3 △ The surgeon marks a new location for the nipple, retrieves it, and stitches it in position.

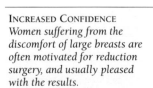

△ BEFORE SURGERY

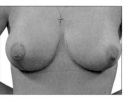

△ AFTER SURGERY

INCREASED CONFIDENCE
Women suffering from the discomfort of large breasts are often motivated for reduction surgery, and usually pleased with the results.

SCARS
Expect some scarring around the areola, in a vertical line down from the areola, and at the base.

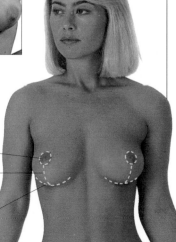

Around areola

From areola to base of breast

Underneath breast

98 BREAST ENLARGEMENT

Enlargement is always achieved with the aid of implants (*Tip 99*), inserted in front of or behind the muscles of the chest wall under the actual breast tissue. The surgery takes at least 1½ hours, and you may need to stay in the hospital for 24 hours to recover from the anesthetic. You should be back to normal in 3–6 weeks.

SILICONE IMPLANTS
The link between silicone implants and cancer, suggested by studies on rats, is unproven. Research into possible problems with silicone implants is ongoing.

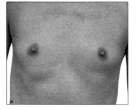

△ BEFORE SURGERY

APPROPRIATE SIZE
Your surgeon will advise you about what would be an appropriate size for your breasts after the operation. Tell him or her what cup size you would like to be – but try to be realistic!

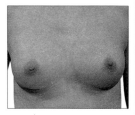

△ AFTER SURGERY

99 IMPLANTS

There are two types of implant: fixed-volume implants (common in cosmetic surgery) and tissue expanders (often used after mastectomy). Both have a textured silicone shell filled with saline (salt in solution) or silicone gel.

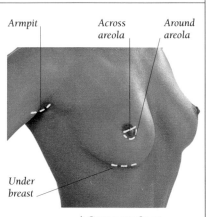

Armpit　*Across areola*　*Around areola*

Under breast

△ **OPERATIVE SITES**
The incision for the operation may be made in the armpit, around or across the areola, or under the breast. Scarring may occur in one of these areas.

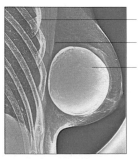

Ribs
Pectoral muscle
Implant

◁ **IMPLANT IN PLACE**
The round, white shape in this mammogram X ray is a silicone implant placed under the glandular tissue of the breast.

100 CORRECTING ASYMMETRY

Even on the same body, no two breasts are the same, and so all women have asymmetry of their breasts to a greater or lesser degree. Some women have breasts that are noticeably asymmetrical, however (*Tip 15*), which makes it difficult to find clothes that fit.

For such women, cosmetic surgery may be worthwhile, and there are three surgical options available:
- enlargement of the smaller breast
- reduction of the larger breast
- a combination of the two.

Whatever you choose, remember that an exact match is unlikely.

101 MASTOPEXY (BREAST-LIFT)

This operation involves removing excess skin and raising the nipple. It can be combined with enlargement if your breasts are small, or reduction if your breasts are very large. Without reduction, mastopexy is not very effective on large breasts because gravity will pull them down. Also, like a face-lift, it is not permanent.

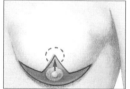

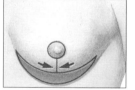

▽ **SCARS**
After the operation, you will be left with some scarring around the areola and under the breast.

1 △ Excess skin and fat, previously marked, are removed from the breast, and the nipple is raised to its new position.

2 △ The skin edges are pulled together and sewn, after which the excess skin is removed from beneath the breast.

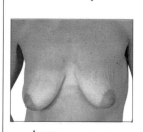

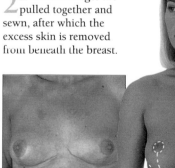

△ BEFORE SURGERY

△ AFTER SURGERY

INDEX

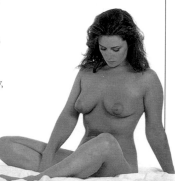

ACKNOWLEDGMENTS

Dorling Kindersley would like to thank Hilary Bird for compiling the index, Richard Hammond for proofreading, Fiona Wild for editorial help, Justine Richards and Maureen Sheerin for picture research, Charlotte Moore for modeling, and Robert Campbell for DTP assistance.

Photography

KEY: t *top*; b *bottom*; c *center*; l *left*; r *right*

The publisher would like to thank the following for their kind permission to reproduce their photographs: Mr. J.D. Frame, St. Andrew's Centre for Plastic Surgery 69bl, 69bc; Dr. Rosalind Given-Wilson, Consultant Radiologist, St. George's Hospital NHS Trust 18cl; Ronald Grant Archive 9tl; Image Bank 43bl, 50bl, 65tr; Nancy Durrell McKenna 31bl; Eleanor Moskovic, The Royal Marsden NHS Trust 18l, 51bl; National Medical Slide Bank 48bl, 48br, 67cl, 68tl, 68tr; Science Photo Library/Chris Bjornberg 54bl /J. Croyle/Custom Medical Stock Photo 54bc /King's College School of Medicine 18cr, 18r, 53tr /Dr. P. Marazzi 35cr, 48bc /Joseph Nettis 59bl /Philippe Plailly 44tr /Breast Screening Unit, King's College Hospital 46bl, 47tr, 47bl / M. Marshall/Custom Medical Stock Photo 68bl; Professor Sir John Sloane, University of Liverpool 52bl, 52bc; Getty Images/Ben Edwards 44cl; Bob Torrez 56bl; Zefa Pictures 11br, 27bl.
All other photographs by Ian Boddy, Andy Crawford, Debi Treloar, Jules Selmes, Clive Streeter.

Illustrations

Tony Graham, Joe Lawrence, Coral Mula, Emma Whiting, Paul Williams.

Models

Helen Bridge & Susannah; James Catto, Claire Farman, & India Rose; Barbara Cogswell, Tracey Coleman, Kerry Cresswell, Aideen Jennings, Patricia Meya, Sheena McFarlane, Mitch Munroe, Wendy Nehorai, Sylvia Newton, Carleena Odumesi, Anna Rizzo, Wendy Rogers, Caroline Sandry, Sharleen Woodsford.

The publisher apologizes to copyright holders and contributors for any unintentional omissions and would be pleased, in such cases, to place an acknowledgment in future editions.

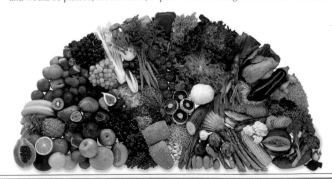